HOLISTIC APPROACHES TO ENHANCING BEAUTY AND SKIN CARE

Expert Guide to Elevate Radiance Natural Techniques for Long-lasting Results And More

DR. CHRIS FRIEDRICH

Disclaimer

This book on Herbal Remedies is intended solely for informational and educational purposes.

The content provided within this book is based on general knowledge and should not be considered as professional advice. The author is not a licensed medical professional, and the information presented here is not intended to diagnose, treat, cure, or prevent any disease.

Readers are advised to consult with qualified healthcare professionals before initiating any herbal remedies or making changes to their existing health regimen. The author and publisher disclaim any responsibility for any adverse effects or consequences resulting from the use of information contained in this book.

It's important to note that the content of this book is not endorsed by any specific platform or affiliated with any product or service.

The author does not receive any compensation or benefits from the promotion of specific herbal products or brands.

Readers should exercise their discretion and judgment when applying the information from this book, and they are encouraged to conduct further research and seek guidance from healthcare professionals to make informed decisions about their health and well-being.

With a focus on the interconnectedness of the mind and body in the pursuit of overall well-being, "Holistic Approaches to Enhancing Beauty and Skin Care" is a thorough guide that delves into the fundamentals of holistic beauty and presents a nuanced understanding of beauty that goes beyond superficial aesthetics. The book starts with a warm welcome and mission statement, setting the stage for an insightful journey into the world of holistic beauty.

The first chapter deftly explains holistic beauty, outlining its tenets and shedding light on the profound influence of the mind-body connection on one's outward appearance. It emphasizes the need to strike a balance between inner and outer beauty to achieve a more genuine and long-lasting radiance. The following chapters delve into various aspects of holistic beauty, beginning with the critical role that nutrition plays in preserving radiant skin. The inclusion of superfoods and the importance of hydration are analyzed, providing readers with actionable advice to improve their skincare routine.

The book then shifts into holistic skincare routines, delving into daily rituals, seasonal adaptations, and mindful practices that contribute to an overall sense of well-being. Herbal remedies and natural ingredients take center stage in the third chapter, unveiling the power of herbs in skincare and providing do-it-yourself herbal skincare recipes. Essential oils are explored for their therapeutic effects on skin health, further enriching the reader's understanding of holistic approaches.

The fifth chapter addresses the complex relationship between emotional health and beauty, highlighting the negative effects of stress on the skin and suggesting holistic approaches to emotional equilibrium. The following chapter addresses the relationship between fitness and beauty, explaining the benefits of exercise and yoga for skin health and presenting holistic fitness regimens as essential elements of attaining a glowing complexion.

Chapter seven explores holistic spa therapies, offering an overview of treatments, guidance for a do-it-yourself holistic spa day at home, and tips for finding reputable holistic spa centers.

Tailored approaches for different skin types are detailed in the eighth chapter, addressing the unique needs of oily, dry, and sensitive skin. Aging gracefully is then addressed in the ninth chapter, emphasizing confidence in embracing the natural aging process and providing holistic anti-aging practices and tips for healthy aging.

"Holistic Approaches to Enhancing Beauty and Skin Care" is a beacon for people seeking a profound and holistic understanding of beauty, providing a roadmap to cultivate enduring radiance from the inside out.

The book's final chapter adopts a forward-looking perspective, examining the relationship between holistic beauty and sustainability.

It advocates for eco-friendly beauty practices, helps readers choose sustainable beauty products, and examines the broader environmental impact of holistic beauty.

First Of All, Greetings And Goals Of The Book

In the constantly changing field of beauty and skincare, a holistic approach has become more popular as people look for all-encompassing and long-lasting ways to improve their well-being.

This book will explore the many facets of holistic beauty and skincare, looking at the different aspects that go into overall skin health and beauty. It will also look at the connections between physical, mental, and environmental factors to give readers a thorough understanding of holistic practices and their significant influence on improving beauty.

The Holistic Method Of Skincare And Beauty

Adopting a holistic perspective entails acknowledging the intricate interplay between lifestyle, nutrition, emotional well-being, and skincare routines. This comprehensive approach recognizes that factors like stress, diet, and emotional balance can significantly influence skin health. By adopting holistic principles, people aim to address the root causes of skin issues instead of merely treating surface-level symptoms. Holistic approaches to beauty and skincare transcend conventional methods by considering the individual as a whole entity instead of focusing solely on external symptoms.

The Advantages Of Holistic Practices For Skin Health

From a physiological perspective, practices like mindful nutrition, stress management, and toxin reduction contribute to improved skin elasticity, hydration, and radiance. Additionally, holistic approaches often lead to a reduction in inflammation, a key factor in many skin conditions. Several benefits for skin health are associated with holistic practices, which emphasize a proactive and preventive approach. Unlike traditional skin care methods, which often target specific concerns, holistic practices work towards creating a balance within the body and mind, fostering overall well-being.

The Effects Of Nutrition On Skin Health

A holistic skin care regimen is incomplete without considering nutrition. The adage "you are what you eat" is especially applicable to the beauty industry. A diet that is rich in nutrients and well-balanced provides the building blocks for healthy skin, impacting factors like collagen production, cell regeneration, and overall skin resilience. This section will discuss the particular vitamins, minerals, and antioxidants that contribute to optimal skin health, discussing their sources and the science behind their effectiveness. It will also explain the relationship between certain dietary patterns, like the Mediterranean diet, and improved skin conditions, providing useful information for those who want to improve their appearance through conscious nutrition.

The Relationship Between Emotional Health And Skin Reflection

Holistic beauty practices are based on the complex relationship between emotional well-being and skin health. Stress, anxiety, and other emotional factors can show up on the skin and cause problems like breakouts, dullness, and early aging. This section will discuss the psych dermatology aspect of the relationship between the mind and the skin. It will also highlight the role that techniques like mindfulness, meditation, and stress reduction strategies play in promoting emotional balance and, ultimately, healthier skin.

Finally, it will discuss the influence of positive emotions on skin radiance and glow, underscoring the significance of holistic practices in fostering a harmonious relationship between mental well-being and external beauty.

Clean Beauty And Toxin Reduction

The concept of holistic skincare goes beyond what we put in our bodies and includes what we put on our skin. Clean beauty highlights the need to use skincare and cosmetic products free of toxic chemicals.

This section will examine common skincare ingredients that may have negative effects on skin health and general well-being as well as the advantages of natural and organic skincare alternatives, giving readers insights into sustainable and non-toxic beauty practices.

The clean beauty movement emerged as a result of growing awareness of the potential long-term consequences of synthetic ingredients.

Skincare And Environmental Factors

The holistic skincare approach acknowledges that environmental factors have an impact on skin health. From pollution and UV radiation to climate variations, external factors can affect the skin's resilience and appearance.

This section will discuss sustainable skincare practices that take environmental impact into account, like eco-friendly packaging and cruelty-free formulations, as well as the science behind how environmental stressors affect the skin, covering topics like oxidative stress, free radical damage, and the role of antioxidants in protection.

Decisions On Lifestyle And Holistic Skincare

Beyond specific practices, lifestyle decisions are critical to the holistic approach to skincare. Sleep, exercise, and daily routines all have a substantial impact on overall well-being, which in turn influences skin health.

This section will examine the science underlying how lifestyle decisions affect skin conditions, from the benefits of regular exercise for skin elasticity to the role of sleep in collagen production.

It will also offer helpful tips for integrating holistic skincare into daily life, such as creating mindful morning and evening routines. Knowing that skincare is holistic helps people to see their lifestyle decisions as essential elements of their journey to beauty enhancement.

Combining Conventional And Contemporary Methods For Holistic Skincare

Case studies and success stories illustrating the efficacy of combining traditional and modern approaches will be presented, illustrating the potential for a synergistic and customized holistic skincare regimen.

 One distinctive feature of holistic skincare is the combination of traditional wisdom and modern scientific advancements.

This section will explore the integration of ancient practices, such as Ayurveda, traditional Chinese medicine, and herbal remedies, with contemporary skincare approaches. By blending time-tested holistic traditions with evidence-based modern practices, individuals can harness the benefits of both worlds.

As the beauty industry continues to change, adopting a holistic perspective not only empowers people to make more conscious and sustainable beauty choices but also contributes to a larger cultural shift towards more mindful and sustainable well-being. By addressing the interconnectedness of various factors, such as nutrition, emotional well-being, environmental considerations, and lifestyle choices, people can embark on a transformative journey toward optimal skin health and beauty.

This book aims to serve as a guide, offering in-depth insights into the science, principles, and real-world applications of holistic skincare.

CHAPTER ONE
UNDERSTANDING HOLISTIC BEAUTY IN

A holistic approach to beauty enhancement looks beyond outward appearances and explores the interplay of multiple factors, recognizing that beauty is more than just skin deep.

Holistic beauty takes into account the whole person—mind, body, and spirit—realizing that external beauty is closely related to internal well-being. According to this perspective, beauty is seen as a mirror of total health and balance, including mental, emotional, and physical components.

The Meaning And Tenets Of Holistic Beauty

Holistic beauty is based on the notion that true beauty arises from a state of harmonious balance between the body, mind, and soul. It deviates from the traditional emphasis on skincare and makeup and instead emphasizes a holistic lifestyle that includes mindfulness, nutrition, stress management, and self-care practices. Holistic beauty recognizes the interdependence of these components and recognizes that radiant skin and a vibrant appearance is the results of a holistic and well-rounded approach to personal well-being. Holistic beauty also aims to address the underlying causes of beauty issues rather than just treating the symptoms.

Beauty's Mind-Body Connection

The core of holistic beauty is a deep understanding of the mind-body connection and how it affects one's appearance. Research backs up the idea that mental and emotional health have a significant impact on skin health and overall beauty. Stress, for example, can physically manifest as skin conditions like acne, eczema, or premature aging. Holistic beauty promotes mental health through practices like yoga, meditation, and mindfulness, acknowledging the positive effects these practices have on skin health.

This paradigm shift emphasizes the significance of maintaining emotional balance for radiant and long-lasting beauty that goes beyond simple cosmetic improvements.

Harmonizing External And Internal Beauty:

While conventional beauty practices tend to emphasize outward appearances, holistic beauty recognizes that nurturing inner well-being contributes to a more sustainable and genuine outward radiance. This includes developing positive self-esteem, fostering self-love, and nurturing a healthy relationship with one's body. By addressing emotional and psychological aspects, holistic beauty aims to create a synergistic relationship between the inner self and external beauty rituals.

This balance is not only aesthetically pleasing but also enhances one's sense of beauty over time.

holistic beauty is a paradigm shift in the way that beauty and skincare are approached. It goes beyond the surface and embraces a comprehensive understanding of beauty as a reflection of overall well-being. The principles of holistic beauty emphasize the interconnectedness of the mind, body, and spirit, acknowledging that true beauty arises from a harmonious balance within.

By addressing the mind-body connection, holistic beauty aims to promote radiant skin and long-lasting beauty from the inside out. At the center of this approach is the balance between inner and outer beauty, motivating people to maintain a holistic lifestyle that integrates mental, physical, and emotional well-being to achieve a more genuine and sustainable attractive appearance.

CHAPTER 2
RADIANT SKIN NUTRITION

The importance of nutrition in skin health cannot be overstated, as the skin is a reflection of our overall health. Different dietary components contribute to the vitality of the skin, influencing factors like elasticity, hydration, and the body's ability to combat oxidative stress.

Researchers and dermatologists emphasize the connection between a balanced diet and skin health, pointing out that deficiencies or imbalances in certain nutrients can manifest as skin issues. A holistic approach to enhancing beauty and skincare recognizes the pivotal role that nutrition plays in achieving and maintaining radiant skin.

Since the skin is a dynamic organ with high metabolic activity, nutrition is important for maintaining skin health.

Vitamins, minerals, and antioxidants are essential for supporting the functions of the skin; for example, vitamin C is necessary for the synthesis of collagen, which is essential for skin elasticity and structure; adequate intake of vitamin E helps shield the skin from oxidative damage; and vitamin A aids in cell turnover and repair.

The holistic approach promotes a well-rounded diet that incorporates a variety of nutrients to address different aspects of skin health.

Superfoods for Beautiful Skin: Superfoods are nutrient-dense foods that provide an abundance of vitamins, minerals, and antioxidants that are good for skin health as well as general health. They are more than just food; they are a proactive way to nourish the body and encourage glowing skin. Skincare experts and nutritionists agree that including superfoods in the diet is a smart move.

Superfoods that are especially well-known for their beneficial effects on skin health include berries, which are high in antioxidants that fight free radicals; fatty fish, such as salmon, which are rich in omega-3 fatty acids that help to hydrate and elasticity the skin; and avocados, which are high in vitamins and essential fatty acids; green tea, with its polyphenols, is known for its anti-inflammatory qualities; and nuts and seeds, which provide skin-friendly nutrients like zinc and selenium.

Eating a diet high in these superfoods is in line with the holistic concept of nourishing the body from the inside out to improve the appearance of the outside.

A holistic approach to skincare emphasizes the importance of internal hydration through sufficient water intake, complementing external skincare routines. Hydration and its Impact on Skin: Water is essential for various physiological processes, including the transportation of nutrients to skin cells, the elimination of waste products, and the regulation of body temperature. Adequate hydration is fundamental for maintaining skin health.

Dehydration can show up as flakiness, dryness, and a generally dull complexion. The holistic approach acknowledges that topical moisturizers alone might not be the best way to address the underlying cause of skin dehydration, so it promotes an internal and external hydration strategy. Drinking enough water, herbal teas, and fruits high in water raises the body's level of hydration, which benefits the skin. In addition, the holistic approach cautions against consuming excessive amounts of dehydrating substances like caffeine and alcohol because of their potential effects on skin moisture.

a holistic approach to improving beauty and skincare highlights the connection between nutrition, superfoods, and hydration to achieve radiant skin. Knowing how nutrition affects skin health highlights the necessity of a well-balanced diet full of vital nutrients. Superfoods are important because they give the body the building blocks it needs to function optimally, addressing a variety of factors like inflammation, oxidative stress, and dehydration. At the same time, realizing the importance of hydration and its impact on the skin calls for an all-encompassing approach that incorporates both internal and external measures. By following these holistic ideas, people can take care of their skin from the inside out, promoting long-term skin health.

CHAPTER 3
NATURAL INGREDIENTS AND HERBAL REMEDIES

The power of natural ingredients and herbal remedies is heavily emphasized in the holistic approach to improving beauty and skincare. Herbal remedies have been used for centuries in skincare practices across cultures because of their therapeutic benefits and low side effects.

The variety of bioactive compounds found in herbs, including antioxidants, anti-inflammatory agents, and antimicrobial substances, work in concert to support skin health and address a variety of dermatological concerns.

When it comes to skincare, herbs are essential for nourishing and revitalizing the skin. Herbs with calming qualities, such as aloe vera, chamomile, and calendula, are effective in reducing skin irritation and redness. Additionally, herbs with strong antimicrobial and anti-inflammatory properties, like turmeric and neem, are useful in treating acne and other skin infections.

Taking a holistic approach to skincare with herbs goes beyond treating symptoms and instead focuses on addressing the underlying causes of skin problems.

DIY herbal skincare recipes make use of readily available herbs like lavender, rosemary, and mint to enable people to make customized skincare products that are tailored to their individual needs. This not only promotes self-reliance but also raises awareness of the ingredients used in skincare, fostering a more conscious and informed approach to beauty practices. DIY herbal skincare recipes further exemplify the holistic approach by encouraging people to actively participate in their skincare routines. This concept recognizes the empowering nature of self-care practices and fosters a deeper connection between individuals and their skincare regimens.

The use of essential oils in skincare is in line with the holistic approach by taking into account not only the physical aspects of skincare but also the emotional and psychological well-being of individuals. Essential oils for Skin Health are concentrated plant extracts that capture the aromatic essence and therapeutic properties of various plants. These oils have gained popularity in skincare because they can address a wide range of skin concerns. For example, tea tree oil is known for its antimicrobial properties, which make it effective in managing acne, while lavender oil is celebrated for its calming and balancing effects on the skin.

, the use of natural ingredients and herbal remedies in skincare represents a holistic paradigm that values the interdependence of physical, emotional, and mental health; it recognizes the various therapeutic qualities of herbs, promotes personal responsibility through do-it-yourself skincare recipes, and capitalizes on essential oils for a customized and all-encompassing skincare routine.

Dietary Methods For Enhanced Skin Brightness

Nutritional approaches to skin radiance highlight the significant influence that nutrition and diet have on skin health and appearance; holistic skincare acknowledges that beauty comes from within and that radiant, healthy skin is the result of a well-balanced, nutrient-rich diet; the complex relationship between nutrition and skin health involves the interaction of multiple vitamins, minerals, antioxidants, and other bioactive compounds that support skin integrity and function.

A varied and nutrient-dense diet is crucial for ensuring an adequate supply of vitamins A, C, and E, which are important for skin health. Vitamin A, which is abundant in foods like sweet potatoes and carrots, promotes cell turnover and helps maintain the integrity of the skin barrier.

Vitamin C, which is strong and antioxidant-rich protects the skin from oxidative stress and supports collagen synthesis. Vitamin E, which is found in nuts and seeds, helps hydrate the skin and protects against UV damage.

The holistic approach to nutritional skincare goes beyond isolated nutrients and promotes a holistic and varied diet to address the multifaceted nature of skin health. Minerals, such as zinc and selenium, are also essential to skin health. Zinc, which is found in foods like pumpkin seeds and chickpeas, plays a role in wound healing and supports the immune system, contributing to overall skin wellness. Selenium, which is present in Brazil nuts and fish, acts as an antioxidant and is involved in the maintenance of skin elasticity.

A diet high in antioxidants can act as a natural defense against external stressors like pollution and UV radiation.

Antioxidant-rich foods are a cornerstone of the nutritional approach to skin radiance.

Rich in antioxidants, foods like berries, green tea, and dark leafy greens help neutralize free radicals, reducing oxidative stress on the skin. The holistic philosophy acknowledges that environmental factors like pollution and UV radiation contribute to skin aging.

Furthermore, the holistic viewpoint on nutritional approaches to skin radiance takes into account the role of hydration in skin health. Sufficient water intake is necessary to preserve skin hydration, elasticity, and overall function.

Skin that is properly hydrated is more resilient and less likely to become dry and irritated.

The holistic approach stresses both the internal and external hydration that is attained through drinking enough water and consuming foods high in water, such as fruits and vegetables.

the holistic approach to skincare recognizes that true skin radiance is a reflection of overall health and well-being and emphasizes the complex relationship between nutrition and skin health. This is achieved by emphasizing a well-rounded, nutrient-dense diet rich in vitamins, minerals, antioxidants, and hydration.

Skincare's Mind-Body Connection

The holistic approach to skincare understands that the mind and body are interconnected and that fostering mental well-being is crucial for achieving optimal skin health. The mind-body connection in skincare represents a holistic paradigm that acknowledges the intricate relationship between mental well-being and the health of the skin.

This concept goes beyond the traditional focus on external skincare practices and acknowledges the impact of stress, emotions, and mental states on the skin's appearance and overall health.

Stress is a major factor that can negatively impact the skin. The release of stress hormones, such as cortisol, can cause inflammation to increase and exacerbate several skin conditions, such as psoriasis, acne, and eczema.

The holistic approach to the mind-body connection in skincare promotes the use of stress-reduction techniques, such as deep breathing exercises, mindfulness exercises, and meditation, to lessen the negative effects of stress on the skin. The holistic approach aims to achieve a harmonious balance between mental and physical well-being by addressing the underlying causes of skin problems.

An integral part of the mind-body connection in skincare is the promotion of emotional well-being. The holistic perspective acknowledges that emotional health is a key determinant of overall well-being and that a positive mindset can positively influence the appearance of the skin.

Emotional well-being also plays a vital role in the holistic approach to skincare. Positive emotions and a healthy mental outlook can contribute to a radiant complexion and improved skin health.

Another facet of the mind-body connection is mindfulness in skincare routines. The holistic approach invites people to be mindful and present during skincare practices.

 This includes appreciating the sensory experience of skincare routines, paying attention to the products used, and developing gratitude for the care that is provided to the skin.

Mindful skincare practices not only improve the efficacy of skincare routines but also support a holistic sense of well-being by encouraging a thoughtful and intentional approach to self-care.

the holistic approach to skincare is best represented by the mind-body connection, which acknowledges the complex relationship between mental and physical health.

Through stress management, emotional support, and mindfulness in skincare regimens, this concept promotes a thorough approach to skincare that transcends superficial treatments and acknowledges the deep connection between the mind and the skin.

CHAPTER 4
HOLISTIC APPROACHES TO SKINCARE PROGRAMS

In the realm of skincare, adopting a holistic approach involves considering the interconnectedness of various aspects of one's life that contribute to overall well-being. Daily Holistic Skincare Rituals form the foundation of this approach, emphasizing a comprehensive routine that extends beyond merely applying topical products. This involves integrating practices that nourish the body from within, such as maintaining a balanced diet, staying hydrated, and engaging in regular exercise. Additionally, recognizing the impact of stress on the skin and incorporating stress-management techniques, such as meditation or yoga, becomes crucial. The holistic skincare routine acknowledges that external factors, like environmental influences, also play a role, prompting individuals to make conscious choices in terms of sun protection and pollution defense. This holistic daily skincare ritual not only aims for external beauty but seeks to promote skin health by addressing internal and external factors simultaneously.

Seasonal Changes and Adaptations: recognizing that skin needs change with the seasons, holistic skincare entails modifying one's skincare regimen by the seasons. For example, in the winter, when skin is typically drier, people may concentrate on heavier moisturizers and treatments that increase hydration; in the summer, when skin is more likely to be oily and sunburned, people may concentrate on lighter formulations and increased sun protection measures. Additionally, holistic skincare recognizes the importance of modifying eating habits to correspond with seasonal changes, realizing that nutritional requirements change with temperature and environmental conditions. This adaptive approach guarantees that skin care is not

Mindfulness in skincare involves being present and attentive during the skincare routine, fostering a positive mindset, and cultivating self-care habits. Stress, a common factor affecting skin conditions, can be mitigated through mindful practices like deep breathing or incorporating aromatherapy into the skincare routine.

Additionally, holistic skincare encourages people to be mindful of product choices, opting for those that align with personal values, such as cruelty-free or environmentally friendly options.

This integration of mindfulness into skincare not only contributes to the psychological well-being of the user but also helps them make more informed decisions about their skin.

Holistic Methods For Improving Beauty

Holistic beauty emphasizes the consumption of whole foods, such as fruits, vegetables, and lean proteins, while minimizing processed and sugary items.

This nutritional approach nourishes the body at the cellular level, fostering a radiant complexion and promoting the longevity of beauty. Holistic beauty goes beyond superficial aesthetics, encompassing various facets that contribute to an individual's overall allure. Nutrition is a cornerstone in this paradigm, acknowledging that beauty radiates from within.

An individual's natural beauty can be enhanced by positive emotions and a balanced mental state; holistic beauty practices often incorporate stress-reduction techniques like mindfulness and meditation to address emotional well-being.

This not only promotes a more youthful appearance but also an inner glow that goes beyond cosmetic enhancements. Holistic beauty also embraces the concept of Emotional Well-Being, acknowledging the profound impact of emotions on one's physical appearance. Chronic stress, for example, can accelerate the aging process and contribute to various skin issues.

Physical activity is another essential element of holistic beauty. Exercise not only improves circulation, which supplies oxygen and nutrients to the skin and fosters a healthy complexion, but it also triggers the release of endorphins, sometimes known as "feel-good" hormones that have a positive impact on mood and, in turn, one's physical appearance. Holistic beauty promotes a variety of physical activities, from aerobic workouts to strength and flexibility training, understanding that each type of exercise adds something special to the improvement of physical attractiveness.

One of the main principles of holistic beauty is environmental consciousness, which emphasizes the relationship between the health of the planet and human well-being. This means that people who practice holistic beauty make thoughtful decisions about the beauty products they use, choosing ones that are cruelty-free, sustainably sourced, and environmentally friendly. Additionally, holistic beauty practices take ethical considerations into account, encouraging the use of products that are in line with values like social responsibility and fair trade.

By recognizing the complex relationships that exist between mental health, physical health, and environmental factors, the holistic approach to skincare and beauty goes beyond traditional paradigms. The foundations of a holistic skincare routine include Daily Holistic Skincare Rituals, Seasonal Changes and Adaptations, and Mindful Skincare Practices. Similarly, the holistic enhancement of beauty includes Nutrition, Emotional Well-Being, Physical Activity, and Environmental Consciousness. Adopting these holistic principles not only fosters overall well-being but also enhances external beauty by promoting mental, physical, and emotional health.

CHAPTER 5
EMOTIONAL WELL-BEING AND BEAUTY

The relationship between emotional well-being and overall health and beauty is complex. When it comes to holistic methods of improving skincare and beauty, it is critical to comprehend and treat emotional well-being. Stress, a prevalent aspect of contemporary life, can have a significant negative impact on the skin and result in several dermatological problems. For this reason, it is important to investigate the relationship between stress and skin health.

The Impact Of Stress On The Skin

Numerous scientific studies have shed light on the complex mechanisms underlying the relationship between stress and skin health. For example, long-term stress can physically affect the skin, exacerbating conditions like psoriasis, eczema, and acne; stress hormones, especially cortisol, can stimulate the sebaceous glands, causing increased oil production and acne; and stress-induced inflammation can aggravate pre-existing conditions and hasten the aging process.

Since the skin is the largest organ, it is a good indicator of one's emotional state. The mind-skin connection is mediated by a complex interaction of immune, endocrine, and neurological factors. Knowing this connection can help you develop practices that support emotional balance and improve the health of your skin.

Strategies For Emotional Harmony

A range of techniques that address the mind-body connection are included in holistic approaches to emotional balance. Mindfulness meditation, for example, is effective in lowering stress and elevating emotional health.

It is an age-old practice that involves developing an impartial awareness of the present moment and can help people better handle stressors. Another technique that promotes emotional resilience and relaxation is yoga, which combines physical postures with breathing exercises and meditation.

Aromatherapy, which uses essential oils to elicit particular emotional responses, is becoming more and more popular for its calming and mood-stabilizing effects. Art therapy, which is based on creative expression, has also shown benefits in reducing stress and improving emotional well-being. Participating in artistic activities gives people an outlet for self-expression, enabling them to process and cope with emotions effectively.

Holistic Views On Beauty And Mental Health

Holistic skincare goes beyond topical treatments to include lifestyle factors that impact mental health. Regular exercise, balanced nutrition, and adequate sleep are essential components of a holistic approach to mental health and beauty.

 Quality sleep, in particular, is crucial for skin regeneration and repair, promoting a radiant complexion. The convergence of mental health and beauty is evident in holistic approaches that emphasize overall well-being rather than merely surface-level aesthetics.

Nutrition is essential for maintaining both the health of the mind and the vitality of the skin. Foods high in antioxidants, like fruits and vegetables, help to counteract free radicals, which reduces oxidative stress and promotes the synthesis of collagen. Omega-3 fatty acids, which are present in fish and flaxseeds, have anti-inflammatory qualities that help with skin conditions and mental health.

Beyond its cardiovascular advantages, exercise elevates mood by releasing endorphins, which are neurotransmitters linked to feelings of happiness and well-being. Including exercise in a holistic beauty regimen not only benefits mental health but also increases circulation, which supports a healthy complexion.

the integration of mental health, emotional well-being, and beauty is a fundamental principle of holistic skincare practices. Understanding how stress affects skin health, implementing emotional balancing techniques, and embracing holistic mental well-being strategies are essential steps toward attaining radiant and long-lasting beauty. By addressing the mind-skin connection, people can take a transformative journey that goes beyond traditional beauty standards, cultivating a harmonious relationship between inner well-being and outer radiance.

CHAPTER 6
BEAUTY AND FITNESS

The relationship between physical activity and skin health is a complex topic that includes various aspects of exercise, yoga, and holistic fitness routines. The intersection of fitness and beauty has gained significant attention in discussions surrounding holistic approaches to enhancing beauty and skincare. This section explores the subtle relationships between fitness and beauty, including the impact of exercise on skin health, the integration of yoga into beauty regimens, and the holistic fitness routines that promote a radiant complexion.

Physical Activity And Skin Health

The relationship between regular physical exercise and skin health is a topic that is gaining more attention in the scientific and beauty communities. Exercise has been demonstrated to have significant effects on general well-being, which includes skin health. Exercise encourages improved blood circulation, which helps skin cells receive oxygen and nutrients. Exercise also releases endorphins, which lowers stress levels and lessens the effects of stress-related skin conditions. Sweating while exercising acts as a natural detoxification process, removing toxins and impurities from the skin. Research has shown that moderate to regular physical activity can contribute to a more youthful appearance by promoting

Yoga With Beautification

Incorporating mindfulness and deep breathing techniques into yoga practices further contributes to skin health by reducing oxidative stress and promoting a calm, balanced complexion.

Beyond its well-documented benefits for mental health and flexibility, yoga is increasingly recognized for its positive impact on skin health.

In addition, certain yoga poses are believed to stimulate blood flow to the face, promoting a natural glow and reducing puffiness. Additionally, yoga's stress-reducing properties can play a crucial role in preventing stress-induced skin issues, like acne and eczema. Furthermore, yoga is an essential component of holistic beauty regimens.

Wholesome Exercise Plans For Stunning Skin

Beyond conventional exercise and yoga, holistic fitness routines are gaining popularity as comprehensive approaches to promoting skin health and beauty. These routines often encompass a combination of physical exercise, mindful practices, and dietary considerations.

The holistic approach recognizes the symbiotic relationship between various lifestyle factors and their impact on skin appearance.

Incorporating elements of cardiovascular exercise, strength training, and flexibility workouts, these routines aim to address different aspects of overall health, reflecting positively on the skin. Additionally, mindfulness practices such as meditation and deep breathing exercises are integral components, as they contribute to stress reduction and promote a sense of balance, further enhancing the skin's natural radiance. The holistic perspective extends beyond physical activities to encompass a holistic lifestyle that includes proper nutrition, hydration, and sufficient rest as essential components for achieving and maintaining beautiful skin.

the holistic approach to improving beauty and skincare includes a thorough comprehension of the relationship between fitness and skin health. Exercise, yoga, and holistic fitness regimens all have unique effects on glowing, healthy skin.

These include the physiological advantages of increased blood circulation and collagen production as well as the psychological benefits of stress reduction and mindfulness.

 These ideas highlight the importance of a holistic lifestyle in attaining long-lasting beauty. As more people look for integrative approaches to well-being, the story of how fitness and skincare are related becomes more compelling. It emphasizes the significance of taking care of both body and mind for a truly holistic beauty experience.

CHAPTER SEVEN
HOLSTIC SPA THERAPIES

The use of holistic spa therapies is one well-known approach in the field of holistic beauty and skincare. Holistic approaches to improving beauty and skincare have gained popularity in recent years, emphasizing a comprehensive and interconnected view of well-being.

This holistic perspective recognizes the intricate relationships between the mind, body, and spirit, and seeks to address beauty and skincare concerns by considering the individual as a whole.

Holistic Spa Treatments

Synopsis of Holistic Spa Services:

Beyond traditional beauty procedures, holistic spa treatments incorporate a variety of elements that address an individual's overall well-being.

These therapies frequently combine traditional spa practices with holistic approaches like aromatherapy, meditation, and energy healing. For example, aromatherapy uses plant-derived essential oils to promote relaxation and emotional well-being, while energy healing techniques like Reiki work to balance the body's energy centers. These holistic spa treatments acknowledge the interdependence of mental, emotional, and physical aspects, making them more comprehensive than traditional beauty and skincare procedures.

At-Home Holistic Spa Day Diy

DIY holistic spa days are becoming more and more popular in today's fast-paced world as an affordable and easy way to prioritize self-care. Setting up a holistic spa experience at home involves carefully choosing skincare products, mindfulness exercises, and relaxation techniques. Natural face masks, essential oils, and herbal teas are frequently used in DIY spa treatments to nourish the skin and encourage relaxation.

Adding mindfulness exercises like meditation and deep breathing exercises further enhances the holistic aspect of the spa day, addressing not only external beauty concerns but also contributing to mental and emotional well-being. DIY holistic spa days encourage people to take charge of their self-care routines, fostering a sense of empowerment and self-reliance.

Locating Centers For Holistic Spas

Finding trustworthy holistic spa centers is crucial for anyone looking for a professional and immersive holistic spa experience. These centers usually offer a variety of treatments that combine traditional spa services with holistic practices, such as holistic facials, body wraps made of natural ingredients, and energy-balancing therapies. It's important to look at the qualifications and experience of the practitioners as well as the types of treatments that are offered when choosing a holistic spa center. Reading reviews and testimonials from previous clients can also give you insight into the efficacy and quality of holistic spa services. Choosing a spa that matches your values and preferences guarantees a more meaningful and personalized experience, which enhances both

holistic spa therapies are a comprehensive approach to skincare and beauty that addresses the interconnected aspects of the mind, body, and spirit. Whether one chooses to learn about holistic spa treatments, create a DIY holistic spa day at home, or choose a reputable holistic spa center, one can adopt these approaches to improve their general well-being. By acknowledging and fostering the harmony between the outside and the inside, holistic spa therapies provide a rejuvenating and transforming experience for those looking to connect with themselves on a deeper level.

CHAPTER 8
HOLISTIC BEAUTY FOR DIFFERENT SKIN TYPES

The term "holistic beauty" refers to a comprehensive skincare approach that takes into account not only external factors but also internal well-being, lifestyle choices, and emotional balance. Customizing holistic care to individual skin types acknowledges that every person's skin is different and has specific needs; it does not prescribe a single product that works for all skin types.

Natural Remedies For Oily Skin

A holistic approach to treating oily skin involves a multimodal approach that combines external skincare practices with internal lifestyle adjustments. External care might involve using non-comedogenic products, incorporating natural ingredients like tea tree oil, which is known for its antibacterial properties, and gently cleansing the skin to remove excess oil without stripping it off. Internally, dietary changes can be crucial, such as cutting back on processed foods and increasing anti-inflammatory foods like omega-3 fatty acids. Finally, managing stress with activities like yoga or meditation is important because stress can worsen oil production.

Complete Skin Care For Dry Skin

Dry skin is defined by a deficiency of moisture, which can cause flakiness, rough texture, and even sensitivity. Holistic care for dry skin is a comprehensive approach to hydrate and nourishing the skin from the inside out. External care for dry skin includes using a mild cleanser, avoiding hot water during cleansing, and incorporating moisturizers with ingredients like hyaluronic acid and glycerin. Hydration is crucial from the inside out, with an emphasis on drinking enough water and including foods high in essential fatty acids. Dietary supplements, such as omega-3, can also aid in skin hydration.

Holistic therapies, such as aromatherapy and stress-reduction techniques, can further improve the general health of people with dry skin.

Integrated Treatment For Sensitive Skin

Since sensitive skin reacts easily to environmental triggers certain skincare products, need to be cared for gently and carefully. To reduce irritation and inflammation, holistic care for sensitive skin entails making thoughtful lifestyle and product choices.

External care involves using fragrance-free and hypoallergenic products, avoiding harsh chemicals, and choosing natural ingredients like chamomile, which has soothing properties. Internal care involves keeping a balanced and anti-inflammatory diet, which may involve avoiding common allergens. Stress management techniques also play a significant role, as stress can exacerbate skin sensitivity. Mindfulness exercises and selecting relaxing activities are further components of a holistic approach.

Fundamentally, holistic beauty for all skin types acknowledges the interaction of internal and exterior elements and provides a customized, long-term skincare regimen that goes beyond band-aid fixes.

Holistic Methods For Youthful And Anti-Aging Skin

Beyond topical remedies, holistic methods to anti-aging address lifestyle decisions, diet, and mental health. Understanding that aging is a multifaceted process impacted by a multitude of factors, a holistic approach seeks to treat these aspects as a whole.

Comprehending The Process Of Aging

Understanding the aging process is essential before exploring holistic anti-aging approaches. Skin aging is caused by both intrinsic (e.g., genetic predisposition) and extrinsic (e.g., sun exposure and lifestyle choices) factors, and holistic care acknowledges that both must be addressed to promote graceful aging.

A Well-Balanced Diet For Youthful Skin

Nutrition is essential for keeping skin youthful from the inside out. A balanced diet high in vitamins, minerals, and antioxidants can help prevent premature aging. Antioxidants, which can be found in fruits and vegetables, fight free radicals that cause aging prematurely. Essential fatty acids, which can be found in foods like salmon and flaxseeds, support skin elasticity and hydration. Collagen-boosting foods, like bone broth, can also be included to improve skin firmness.

Lifestyle Decisions And Age-Reduction

Holistic anti-aging encompasses lifestyle decisions that support general health, which in turn benefits the skin indirectly. For example, frequent exercise improves blood circulation, which facilitates the delivery of nutrients to skin cells and the elimination of toxins. Adequate sleep is also important because it permits the skin to undergo repair and regeneration. Refusing to smoke and drinking too much alcohol is also important because these behaviors contribute to premature aging by depleting the body of essential nutrients and hastening the breakdown of collagen.

Healthy Minds And Aging

The holistic understanding of the interconnectedness of body and mind is reflected in the integration of mental well-being into anti-aging strategies. The mind-body connection is a fundamental tenet of holistic approaches to anti-aging. Chronic stress can accelerate the aging process, leading to the development of fine lines and wrinkles. Holistic care involves the incorporation of stress-reducing practices like mindfulness meditation, yoga, and deep breathing exercises. These practices not only contribute to mental well-being but also have tangible effects on skin health by reducing inflammation and promoting a more youthful complexion.

holistic methods of anti-aging involve a multimodal strategy that extends beyond topical treatments, tackling lifestyle, mental health, and nutrition. This all-encompassing approach seeks to support not just young skin but also general health and wellness.

Sustainable Environmental Practices And Holistic Beauty

As environmental consciousness has grown, holistic beauty has expanded its tenets to take sustainability into account. Acknowledging the relationship between one's health and the health of the planet, holistic beauty practices prioritize ethical and sustainable decisions over environmental impact.

Eco-Friendly And Pure Beauty Products

Clean beauty practices are supported by holistic beauty, which emphasizes the use of natural, non-toxic ingredients that are good for the skin and the environment. Products with minimal packaging, recyclable materials, and sustainable sourcing practices are chosen, and eco-friendly packaging options like glass or recycled materials are in line with the holistic principle of taking the larger environmental effects of beauty routines into consideration.

Eco-Friendly Skincare Techniques

Reusable and eco-friendly skincare tools, like bamboo facecloths or reusable cotton rounds, align with the holistic ethos of minimizing the ecological footprint of beauty rituals. Additionally, choosing products with refill options promotes a circular and sustainable approach to skincare. Beyond product selection, holistic beauty encourages sustainable skincare practices that reduce waste and environmental impact. This may involve adopting a minimalist approach to skincare, prioritizing multi-use products, and avoiding excessive consumption.

Fair Trade Policies And Ethical Purchasing

Complying with the holistic principle of fostering interconnected well-being, holistic beauty acknowledges that beauty should not come at the expense of environmental degradation or exploitation of communities. By prioritizing products with ethically sourced and fair-trade ingredients, the beauty industry ensures that it positively impacts the well-being of communities involved in production.

Handmade Cosmetics With Repurposed Materials

A sustainable and holistic approach that values resourcefulness and environmental responsibility, holistic beauty embraces the do-it-yourself (DIY) mentality, encouraging people to make their skincare products using natural, locally sourced ingredients. This minimizes the carbon footprint associated with manufacturing and transportation, as well as reliance on mass-produced products. Upcycling, repurposing, and finding new uses for existing beauty containers are also aspects of this approach.

holistic beauty and environmental sustainability are related ideas that highlight the significance of making thoughtful decisions about beauty practices. People can align their beauty routines with a holistic approach that promotes both their well-being and the health of the planet by taking into account the environmental impact of products, adopting sustainable skincare practices, and placing a high value on ethical sourcing.

CHAPTER 9
HOLISTIC STRATEGIES FOR GRACEFUL AGING

Accepting Aging With Self-Assurance

One of the cornerstones of holistic beauty and skincare is embracing aging with confidence. In a culture that frequently places a premium on youthful appearances, cultivating a positive attitude toward the natural aging process becomes imperative. This concept highlights the acceptance of aging as a natural and inevitable part of life, promoting mental well-being and self-esteem. Age-neutral confidence in one's appearance radiates a unique beauty that surpasses conventional standards. Proponents of this approach encourage people to celebrate the wisdom and experiences that come with aging, cultivating a mindset that values inner beauty and self-assurance.

Comprehensive Anti-Aging Techniques

Holistic anti-aging practices constitute a comprehensive and integrated approach to skincare that goes beyond superficial treatments. Instead of merely targeting surface-level concerns, holistic anti-aging seeks to address the root causes of aging, considering both internal and external factors. This approach recognizes the interconnectedness of various aspects of health, including nutrition, stress management, sleep patterns, and emotional well-being.

Holistic anti-aging practices often involve a combination of lifestyle adjustments, incorporating a balanced diet rich in antioxidants, regular physical activity, mindfulness techniques, and adequate rest. By promoting overall health and wellness, these practices aim to slow down the aging process from within, leading to sustained and natural improvements in skin quality and appearance. Additionally, holistic anti-aging may include alternative therapies such as acupuncture, herbal remedies, and facial exercises, further emphasizing the integration of mind, body, and spirit.

Suggestions For A Healthier Aging Population:

Tips for healthy aging encompass a diverse range of practices that contribute to overall well-being and longevity. From a skincare perspective, these tips extend beyond the conventional and delve into lifestyle choices that impact the aging process. Adequate hydration is emphasized as a cornerstone, promoting skin elasticity and resilience.

Regular physical activity is advocated not only for its cardiovascular benefits but also for its role in promoting circulation, which is crucial for a healthy complexion. Furthermore, a nutrient-rich diet, comprising vitamins, minerals, and antioxidants, is underscored for its positive effects on skin health. In the context of healthy aging, stress management techniques, such as meditation and mindfulness, play a vital role in preventing premature aging and maintaining a youthful glow. Additionally, prioritizing quality sleep is considered integral to the regeneration and repair processes that occur during rest, contributing significantly to skin rejuvenation. Altogether, these tips for healthy aging form a holistic framework that addresses the multifaceted nature of the aging process, emphasizing the importance of a balanced and mindful approach to skincare and overall well-being.

holistic approaches to improving beauty and skincare are complex and go beyond traditional methods. Embracing aging with confidence entails a mental shift toward accepting and celebrating life's natural course, promoting mental health and self-worth. Holistic anti-aging practices adopt a comprehensive approach, addressing internal and external factors that contribute to aging, stressing lifestyle modifications and alternative therapies. Practical advice is offered by tips for healthy aging, which integrate elements like hydration, nutrition, physical activity, stress management, and sleep into a comprehensive framework for preserving overall well-being. Collectively, these ideas constitute a holistic paradigm that acknowledges the interconnectedness of

CHAPTER 10
SUSTAINABILITY AND HOLISTIC BEAUTY

Holistic beauty is a comprehensive approach to beauty enhancement that incorporates physical, mental, and environmental aspects.

It acknowledges the interdependence of different aspects of our lives and highlights the significance of balance for overall health. A fundamental feature of holistic beauty is its dedication to sustainability, which recognizes the negative environmental effects of beauty practices and promotes eco-friendly alternatives.

Eco-Friendly Beauty Techniques

A variety of sustainable decisions that lessen the adverse effects of beauty routines on the environment are included in eco-friendly beauty practices.

These decisions include cutting back on the use of single-use plastic, selecting products with minimal packaging, and integrating energy-efficient practices into beauty routines. For example, people can choose to use reusable and biodegradable beauty tools, like bamboo brushes and wooden applicators, to reduce waste generation. Water-conserving measures, such as taking shorter showers and turning off the taps while using skincare products, are also considered to be part of eco-friendly beauty practices.

Moreover, the notion of eco-friendly beauty encompasses the mitigation of detrimental emissions and pollution linked to the processes involved in the manufacturing of beauty products. Businesses that embrace environmentally friendly production techniques and employ renewable energy sources are indicative of their dedication to ecologically responsible practices.

This comprehensive strategy compels customers to take into account the entire lifecycle of products, from the procurement of raw materials to their eventual disposal, thereby fostering a more sustainable and conscientious beauty industry.

Selecting Eco-Friendly Cosmetics

Choosing sustainable beauty products is a key component of holistic beauty. Sustainable beauty products are those that emphasize cruelty-free testing, ethical sourcing, and environmentally friendly packaging. Cruelty-free testing guarantees that products are developed without injuring animals, encouraging a compassionate and responsible approach to beauty. Finally, environmentally friendly packaging minimizes waste by using recyclable materials and minimizing excess packaging.

Customers are the primary force behind the demand for sustainable beauty products, which forces the beauty industry to adopt morally and environmentally sound practices. The emergence of certifications like cruelty-free and organic labels suggests that consumers are becoming more conscious of the ethical and environmental consequences of the cosmetic decisions they make. This move toward sustainability is a reflection of a broader cultural recognition of the relationship between one's health and the health of the planet.

Holistic Beauty's Effects On The Environment

The environmental impact of holistic beauty goes beyond individual practices to affect the beauty industry as a whole. With consumers placing a higher value on sustainability, beauty companies are being forced to reconsider their production methods, suppliers of ingredients, and environmental impact overall. This change has prompted the development of green technologies, like innovative eco-friendly packaging and sustainable ingredient substitutes, which help to create a more earth-conscious and responsible beauty industry.

Furthermore, the holistic approach to beauty places a strong emphasis on education and awareness of the environmental effects of decisions made in the beauty industry. Sustainable beauty practices involve choosing products wisely, being aware of their life cycles, and actively supporting eco-friendly businesses. As a result of this increased awareness, consumers feel more responsible, which in turn motivates them to push for changes in the beauty industry and encourages a community commitment to environmental conservation.

As the beauty industry continues to evolve, embracing holistic and sustainable practices is essential for promoting a healthier and more harmonious relationship between individuals and the planet. Holistic beauty and sustainability are intrinsically linked concepts that highlight the need for a comprehensive approach to beauty that considers the interconnectedness of personal well-being and environmental health. Individuals can contribute to a more responsible and sustainable beauty industry through eco-friendly beauty practices, the choice of sustainable beauty products, and an awareness of the impact on the environment.

CONCLUSION
Review Of The Principles Of Holistic Beauty

This in-depth investigation of holistic methods for improving beauty and skincare reveals that a holistic viewpoint transcends traditional beauty regimens, emphasizing the interdependence of mind, body, and spirit. Holistic beauty principles stress equilibrium between external skincare routines and internal health, recognizing that genuine beauty arises from the balance of physical, mental, and emotional well-being.

The principles covered include proper nutrition for the body, embracing mindful practices, and utilizing natural skincare remedies. This synopsis highlights the significance of embracing a holistic mindset to attain sustainable and holistic beauty results.

Motivation To Lead A Holistic Life

Encouraging holistic living is essential to the quest for improved skincare and beauty. Holistic living is defined as a way of life that places an emphasis on total well-being and recognizes the mutually reinforcing relationship between an individual's internal and external states.

Taking a holistic approach entails developing healthy habits like regular exercise, enough sleep, and stress management. It also encourages people to make conscious decisions in their daily lives, such as choosing nourishing foods and implementing mindfulness practices.

Acknowledging Beauty Internally

The notion of embracing beauty from the inside out highlights the intrinsic relationship between internal health and outward appearance.

It also challenges the traditional belief that beauty is only skin-deep, emphasizing that radiant skin is a reflection of a well-nourished body, a balanced mind, and a harmonious spirit. Individuals can support the body's natural processes and promote healthy skin from the inside by putting nutrition and hydration first.

Adopting mindfulness practices, such as stress reduction and meditation, further enhances overall well-being and radiance. Cultivating self-love and acceptance is encouraged by the idea that true beauty transcends physical appearance.

The investigation of holistic approaches to improving beauty and skincare has illuminated the interdependence of physical, mental, and emotional well-being.

A summary of holistic beauty principles emphasizes the significance of a balanced and integrated approach, stressing the relationship between internal health and outward appearance. Promoting holistic living catalyzes positive change, pushing people to make lifestyle decisions that promote overall well-being. Lastly, accepting beauty from the inside out denotes a paradigm shift, realizing that true radiance arises when people prioritize self-care, nourishment, and mindfulness.

www.ingramcontent.com/pod-product-compliance
Lightning Source LLC
Chambersburg PA
CBHW061004260726

48661CB00005B/2050